VAGUS NERVE

Accessing the Healing Power of the Vagus Nerve for Anxiety

Michael Johnson

© Copyright 2021 - All rights reserved.

This document is geared towards providing exact and reliable information in regards to the topic and issue covered. The publication is sold with the idea that the publisher is not required to render accounting, officially permitted, or otherwise, qualified services. If advice is necessary, legal or professional, a practiced individual in the profession should be ordered.

- From a Declaration of Principles which was accepted and approved equally by a Committee of the American Bar Association and a Committee of Publishers and Associations.

In no way is it legal to reproduce, duplicate, or transmit any part of this document in either electronic means or in printed format. Recording of this publication is strictly prohibited and any storage of this document is not allowed unless with written permission from the publisher. All rights reserved.

The information provided herein is stated to be truthful and consistent, in that any liability, in terms of inattention or otherwise, by any usage or abuse of any policies, processes, or directions contained within is the solitary and utter responsibility of the recipient reader. Under no circumstances will any legal responsibility or blame be held against the publisher for any reparation, damages, or monetary loss due to the information herein, either directly or indirectly.

Respective authors own all copyrights not held by the publisher.

The information herein is offered for informational purposes solely, and is universal as so. The presentation of the information is without contract or any type of guarantee assurance.

The trademarks that are used are without any consent, and the publication of the trademark is without permission or backing by the trademark owner. All trademarks and brands within this book are for clarifying purposes only and are the owned by the owners themselves, not affiliated with this document.

CHAPTER 1. INTRODUCTION TO VAGUS NERVE 5
1.1 STRUCTURE AND FUNCTION 6
1.2 SURGICAL AND CLINICAL CONSIDERATIONS 9
1.3 NEUROANATOMY OF VAGUS NERVE 12
CHAPTER 2. VAGUS NERVE ROLE IN INTESTINAL INFLAMMATION, MOOD AND APPETITE CONTROL 18
2.1 VAGAL ANATOMY 20
2.2 EFFECTS OF DIET AND OBESITY ON VAGUS NERVE FUNCTIONS 23
2.3 MODULATION AND INFLAMMATION OF VAGAL AFFERENTS 28
2.4 PRECLINICAL EVIDENCE OF INTESTINAL INFLAMMATORY DISORDERS 36
2.5 EVIDENCE AND TREATMENT IN HUMANS 41
CHAPTER 3. ROLE OF VAGUS NERVE AS MODULATOR OF THE BRAIN 46
3.1 INTRODUCTION 47
3.2 ROLE OF VAGUS NERVE IN AUTONOMIC NERVOUS SYSTEM 49
3.3 VAGUS NERVE HELPS IN INTESTINAL IMMUNE HOMEOSTASIS 56
3.4 NEURAL MECHANISM 58
3.5 VAGUS NERVE AND TREATMENT OF DEPRESSION 62
CONCLUSION 67

Chapter 1. Introduction to Vagus Nerve

The vagus nerve, or CN X, the 10th cranial nerve, is a nerve that serves various significant capacities. While most of the fascicles work in parasympathetic action, the vagus nerve likewise contains physical tactile, instinctive tangible, and branch like engine filaments. In Latin, vagus signifies, "meandering, wandering." The vagus nerve is accordingly named on the grounds that it follows a mind boggling course all through the body to innervate a few organs; strands begin from the dorsal engine core and core ambiguous in the ventral medulla oblongata of the brainstem, with terminal branches arriving at the splenic flexure of the colon. A basic division during the nerve's course from rostral to caudal happens as it enters the stomach cavity: it parts into a foremost trunk and a back trunk. The primary and utilitarian properties of the foremost trunk, alongside its significant careful and clinical contemplations, will be analyzed in this article.

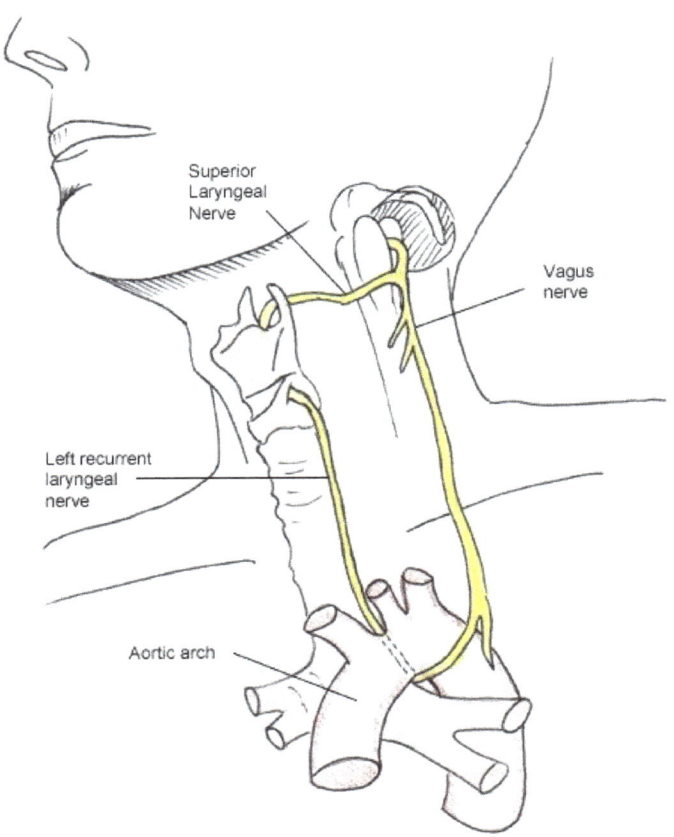

1.1 Structure and Function

Four cores situated at different levels of the medulla house cell collections of the vagus nerve: the dorsal core, which serves parasympathetic capacity to the heart, lungs, and gastrointestinal parcel through broad instinctive efferent strands; the core ambiguous, which is liable for unique instinctive efferent movement and houses cell bodies for the vagus nerve, yet in addition for the 10th and eleventh cranial nerves; the singular core, which gets general instinctive afferent innervation from the carotid body and sinus by means of cranial nerve nine, general instinctive afferent data from the aortic bodies and Sino atrial hub of the heart, just as exceptional instinctive afferent data (i.e., taste) from the foremost 66% of the tongue.

The vagus nerve legitimate is shaped from different rootlets as it rises out of the cranial vault through the jugular foramen. After its development, two tactile ganglia structure: these are the unrivaled ganglion and sub-par ganglion. These ganglia house the cell assortments of the tangible neurons answerable for the vagus nerve's afferent action.

As the vagus nerve enters the stomach pit through the esophageal break, it parts into a foremost trunk and a back trunk. The foremost trunk is basically liable for gastrointestinal parasympathetic innervation to the lesser curve of the stomach, the pylorus, the biliary device, and the gallbladder.

Embryology

The vagus nerve's embryological beginnings can be followed back to exceptional instinctive, just as broad instinctive afferent and efferent cores that emerge from the myelincephalon.

From the 6th week, it is feasible to recognize the cranial nerves, among which is the 10th cranial nerve. There is a cozy connection between the advancement of the vagus nerve and the enteric framework. The embryological flyer included is the ectoderm.

Blood Supply and Lymphatics

An unequivocal vein, the vagal corridor, gives the essential blood supply to the vagus nerve. This corridor tracks on the front surface of the nerve and is at significant danger during a few surgeries.

The Broncho esophageal corridor supplies the vagus nerve with a branch in the mediastinum, to one side in the sub aortic district. Also, in the mediastina area, the vagus nerve can be vascularized by supply routes from the aortic curve, from a first intercostal vein, and second rate thyroid conduit.

The veins that influence the vagus nerve at the level of the mediastinum are the inward thoracic vein from the foremost region and the thoracic intercostal veins from the back region.

Nerves

Significant parts of the vagus nerve include: the predominant laryngeal nerve, which has two branches, the interior laryngeal nerve (in danger with territorial lymphadenopathy or injury), and the outer laryngeal nerve (in danger during prevalent thyroid course ligation); and the repetitive laryngeal nerve (in danger as it folds over the aortic curve on the left-gave side; thusly, aortic curve pathology, like an aneurysm of any sort, jeopardizes this nerve. It can likewise be harmed during patent ductus arteriosus fix, just as perioperative during ligation of the close by sub-par thyroid conduit.

The vagus nerve parts into two trunks: the foremost and back vagal trunks. The foremost trunk, which gets critical commitments from the left vagus nerve more so than the right, branches into: a hepatic branch, which supplies the liver, gallbladder, and biliary mechanical assembly; a celiac branch, which contributes parasympathetic filaments to the celiac plexus; and various front gastric branches, the most average of which courses along the lesser ebb and flow of the stomach. The pylorus and proximal duodenum get innervation from the foremost and back nerves of Latarjet, which are the two branches off of the front vagal trunk.

Muscles

A few muscles get innervation from the vagus nerve: the center and mediocre pharyngeal constrictor muscles, which are answerable for section of food boluses; the palatoglossus, which hoists the back part of the tongue on gulping; and the laryngeal muscles, the aryepiglottic, thyroarytenoid, arytenoid, sidelong and back cricoarytenoid, which are innervated by the repetitive laryngeal nerve. The whole length of the throat is likewise the beneficiary of engine innervation.

The vagus nerve innervates the crural space of the stomach (where the throat passes or esophageal break). The 10th cranial nerve innervates the suspensory muscle of the duodenum or musculus suspensorius duodeni.

Physiologic Variants

In an investigation of 50 analysis, Jackson et al. talked about anatomical variations of the vagus nerve in the space of the distal throat and stomach. From their examples, they tracked down that the left vagus nerve offered a greater number of filaments to the foremost vagal trunk than did the right, but the correct vagus offered more branches generally speaking.

In their investigation of the spreading example of the foremost vagal trunk, they discovered four unmistakable kinds of examples: in one example (type A, 33 examples), the front trunk turned into a solitary trunk over the stomach, and consequently went through the stomach; in another variety (type B, 14 examples), the front vagal trunk was likewise framed over the stomach, as in the past variety, yet split into two particular branches not long prior to experiencing the stomach; a third sort (type C, two examples), in which a solitary trunk didn't shape until the trunks arrived at the stomach; and a last sort (type D, one example), in which the specialists noticed no single trunks over the stomach.

1.2 Surgical and Clinical Considerations

Fundoplication

The foremost vagal trunk and its branches are at significant danger during medical procedures implying the distal throat, stomach, proximal duodenum, biliary plot, and gallbladder. One such medical procedure is the fundoplication, frequently showed in great careful up-and-comers who experience the ill effects of gastro esophageal reflux sickness headstrong to clinical treatment.

Examiners have explored different avenues regarding cutting off the hepatic part of the foremost vagal trunk while playing out a fundoplication to decide the post-usable impacts on the capacity of the gallbladder. This branch falling off the front vagal trunk innervates the liver, biliary contraption, and gives engine innervation to the gallbladder (i.e., gallbladder contractile capacity). Purdy contemplated this in light of the fact that laparoscopic fundoplications were considered actually simpler with the cutting of this branch, however restricted information about postoperative consequences for general gallbladder engine work was accessible. They refer to a Finnish specialist, Dr. M. Paakkonen, who modified the method of dealing with the hepatic branch during fundoplications in 2001. Patients who had fundoplications done when this date got indication surveys; from these patients, 19 were examined further in two particular gatherings. Specifically, the volume of the gallbladder and gallbladder discharge division after a greasy feast (estimated by ultrasound) were of significance, just as the serum convergences of soluble phosphatase, alanine aminotransferase, complete bilirubin, and amylase. The agents noticed no critical contrast in manifestations or PRN utilization of prescription between the two gatherings.

A typical and deplorable post-usable symptom of this methodology is fart. A report distributed in September of 2019 by Cockbain researched the rate of post-usable fart in patients who went through essential laparoscopic fundoplication. The examination entitled Flatulence after Anti-reflux Treatment

(FAART) recognized select patients who had this system accomplished for indicative gastro esophageal reflux infection stubborn to clinical treatment from 1999 and 2009, and investigated occurrence of tooting at follow-up. At a development of 8 to 15 years post-operation, 85% of patients announced extreme fart. The investigation likewise presumed that tooting was to be sure more regrettable in patients who had an all-out fundoplication rather than the individuals who went through a halfway fundoplication. Albeit the rate in this populace was high, the general effect on day by day life was little.

Gastro paresis

A condition characterized by postponed gastric exhausting, gastro paresis presents in patients with queasiness, heaving, swelling, tooting, early satiety, and loss of hunger. The component of the postponed gastric discharging seen here is believed to be intervened by an aggravation in the strength and timing of standard gastric contractility. While different reasons for postponed gastric purging might be identified with a mechanical impediment, gastro paresis is generally either idiopathic, a dreaded entanglement of diabetes mellitus because of autonomic neuropathy or even a consequence of iatrogenic harm during stomach a medical procedure. The main line pharmacological specialist utilized for gastro paresis is metoclopramide, a dopamine receptor foe that has pro kinetic properties. Second-line specialists incorporate erythromycin and cisapride.

A grounded reason for gastro paresis in the diabetic patient populace is an autonomic neuropathy of the vagus nerve. At the point when the parasympathetic capacity to the proximal foregut is undermined, specifically, gastric fundic and antral engine movement, gastric substance can't progress at a calculable rate, bringing about the ordinary indications patients experience. Patients with diabetes and poor glycemic control can encounter neuropathies of an assortment of nerves, just as autonomic neuropathies, either cardiovascular or gastrointestinal, which can end up being particularly troubling.

An investigation distributed in 2005 by Moldovan et al. examined diabetic gastro paresis in 36 patients by means of ultrasonography methods. Thirteen patients with diabetes mellitus type 1 were in the investigation test (HbA1c is equivalent to 8.1), and 23 with diabetes mellitus type 2 contained the remainder of the subjects (HbA1c is equivalent to 9.7). Zeroing in explicitly on autonomic causes, the examiners further split patients into bunches dependent on their sort of diabetes, and whether they were found to have ordinary gastric purging or deferred gastric discharging. In the gathering of type 1 diabetics, they saw that half with typical gastric exhausting tried strangely for parasympathetic neuropathy; in those with postponed gastric discharging, 71.5% tried positive for parasympathetic irregularities. In the gathering included sort 2 diabetics, the accompanying outcomes were accomplished: 46.5% with ordinary gastric purging showed distorted parasympathetic capacity, and 75% with deferred gastric discharging uncovered parasympathetic anomalies.

1.3 Neuroanatomy of Vagus Nerve

The vagus nerve (cranial nerve [CN] X) is the longest cranial nerve in the body, containing both engine and tangible capacities in both the afferent and efferent respects. The nerve ventures broadly all through the body influencing a few organ frameworks and districts of the body, like the tongue, pharynx, heart, and gastrointestinal framework. Due to the wide dispersion of the nerve all through the body, there are a few clinical relationships of the vagus nerve.

The vagus nerve has its starting point in the medulla oblongata and exits the skull through the jugular foramen. There are two ganglia on the vagus nerve (predominant and sub-par) as it leaves the jugular foramen; the spinal embellishment nerve (CN XI) joins the vagus nerve only distal to the sub-par ganglion.

The beginning of cell bodies for the vagus nerve starts from the core uncertain; the dorsal engine core of X, predominant ganglion of X, and the sub-par ganglion of X. The nerve filaments from the core uncertain are efferent, unique instinctive (ESV) strands which help to intervene gulping and phonation. Strands beginning from the dorsal engine core of X are efferent, general instinctive (EGV) filaments which give the compulsory muscle control of organs it innervates (heart, aspiratory, esophageal) and innervation to organs all through the gastrointestinal parcel. Unrivaled ganglion of X gives afferent general substantial innervation to the outside ear and tympanic film. The substandard ganglion of X gives afferent general instinctive strands to the carotid and aortic bodies; the efferent filaments of this nerve travel to the core tractus solitarius; the sub-par ganglion likewise gives taste sensation to the pharynx and transfers this data to the core tractus solitarius.

The vagus nerve proceeds by voyaging poorly inside the carotid sheath where it is found back and horizontal to the interior and basic carotid corridors, and average to the inner jugular vein. The correct vagus nerve goes anteriorly to the subclavian corridor and afterward back to the innominate conduit; it makes its plummet into the thoracic cavity by going to one side of the windpipe, and back to the hilum on the right, moving medially to frame the esophageal plexus with the left vagus nerve. The left vagus nerve ventures out anteriorly to the subclavian course and enters the thoracic hole wedged between the left normal carotid and subclavian corridors; it at that point slips posteriorly to the phrenic nerve and back to one side lung, at that point goes medially towards to the throat framing the esophageal plexus with the correct vagus nerve.

There are four parts of the vagus nerve inside the neck: pharyngeal branches, unrivaled laryngeal nerve, repetitive laryngeal nerve, and the prevalent heart nerve. The pharyngeal nerve branches emerge from the substandard ganglion of CN X containing both tangible and engine strands. These strands structure the pharyngeal plexus–parts of this plexus innervate the pharyngeal and sense of taste muscles (with the exception of the tensor palatine muscle); the pharyngeal plexus additionally supplies the innervation to the intercarotid plexus which intervenes data from the carotid body.

The unrivaled laryngeal nerve goes between the outer and inside carotid supply routes; the nerve isolates into inner and outside branches close to the level of the hyoid. The interior laryngeal nerve goes through the thyrohyoid layer entering the larynx. The outer part ventures distally with the prevalent thyroid vessels. The outside parcel supplies the cricothyroid muscle, while the inward branch supplies the mucosa better than the glottis.

The privilege repetitive laryngeal nerve's strands branch from the vagus nerve close to the privilege subclavian supply route, venturing out superiorly to enter the larynx between the cricopharyngeus muscle and the throat. The left intermittent laryngeal nerve at that point circles around the aortic curve distal to the ligamentum arteriosus and afterward enters the larynx. The entirety of the laryngeal musculatures gets supply through the intermittent laryngeal nerve aside from the cricothyroid muscle (provided by the laryngeal nerve).

While the vagus nerve is inside the carotid sheath, it emits the unrivaled cardiovascular nerve and is related with parasympathetic strands and goes to the heart. The vagus nerve radiates front and back bronchial branches in which the foremost branches are along the front lung framing the front pneumonic plexus, while the back branches structure the back aspiratory plexus.

Esophageal parts of the vagus nerve are foremost and back and structure the esophageal plexus. The left vagus is foremost to the throat; the correct vagus is back. Gastric branches supply the stomach; celiac branches (predominantly got from the correct vagus nerve) supply the pancreas, spleen, kidneys, adrenals, and small digestive tract. The vagus nerve emerges from the fourth branchial curve; this curve is likewise answerable for the advancement of the pharyngeal and laryngeal muscles, the laryngeal ligaments, the aortic curve, and subclavian course.

The center meningeal conduit supplies the intracranial blood supply to the vagus nerve. The extracranial blood supply is from the basic carotid corridor, interior carotid conduit, second rate thyroid course, outer carotid vein, a back meningeal corridor, inward thoracic conduits, bronchial veins, and esophageal supply routes. The vagal framework is engaged with directing the withdrawal of lymphatic (containing actin) cells. The vagus nerve includes branches inside the neck; these branches are the pharyngeal branches, predominant laryngeal nerves, repetitive laryngeal nerves, and unrivaled heart nerves. The design and capacity of these nerves were depicted previously.

The vagus nerve has a few filaments that innervate the striated muscles of the larynx and pharynx; there are two special cases: the stylopharyngeus muscle (CNIX) and the tensor veli palatini muscle (V3). The vagus nerve innervates one muscle of the tongue: palatoglossus muscle–its capacity is to hoist the back segment of the tongue. The outside part of the prevalent laryngeal nerve supplies the cricothyroid muscle. The pharyngeal parts of the vagus supply: levator veli palatini, salpingopharyngeus, palatopharyngeus, and the uvula.

Repetitive laryngeal nerves innervate the natural muscles of the larynx, with the exception of the cricothyroid muscle (the outer part of the predominant laryngeal nerve). The repetitive laryngeal nerve has two branches preceding embedding into the larynx; the stretching is regularly substandard compared to the cricoid ligament; in any case, there are cases when there are multiple branches, and accordingly are called esophageal branches.

There are a few varieties of the non-intermittent vagus nerve. Thought for the parts of the intermittent laryngeal nerve is basic during medical procedure of the thyroid organ. On account of the nearness of the thyroid organ and the parts of the repetitive laryngeal nerve, proposals are for keeping up all nerves in this locale except if there is a tradeoff of the actual nerve by harm.

The repetitive laryngeal nerve might be harmed during a cervical esophagectomy, during the evacuation of a pharyngoesophageal diverticulum or a gastro esophageal anastomosis in the wake of playing out the trans-hiatal esophagectomy. In the diverticulum extraction and the anastomosis, the repetitive laryngeal nerve is lesion from pressure applied by retractors in the working room. Harm should be possible to the outer laryngeal nerve at the hour of ligation of the prevalent thyroid corridor during a thyroidectomy.

The vagus nerve is usually tried clinically in formation with the glossopharyngeal nerve on account of their evident impacts that are in many cases dependent upon another. A patient is frequently approached to open their mouth and say 'ah,' this should cause rise of the uvula. In the event that there is an injury, the uvula moves from the deadened side. Gag reflex ought not to be utilized as a clinical test as there can be a reciprocal loss of the gag reflex in a solid patient. In the event that a patient is noted to have roughness during the actual test, this should show the need to test the vocal strings in the patient; if there is dryness with an ordinary gag reflex and palatal height, this demonstrates a sore of the repetitive laryngeal nerve.

Vagus nerve incitement was made as a way to arrive at a halfway found neurological constructions by insignificantly intrusive methods. In the ordinary vagus nerve incitement method, a gadget is embedded precisely under the skin in the chest, and electrical wires interface with the left vagus nerve (left utilized more frequently than right, as the correct vagus nerve is bound to have branches to the heart). Vagus nerve incitement is supported to treat epilepsy and melancholy; be that as it may, with the wide dissemination of the vagus nerve all through the body, incitement is being investigated for different purposes like the treatment of heftiness.

Incitement of the larynx gives reflexes including hack, apnea, and consequences for the cardiovascular framework like bradycardia and hypotension. Focal sores of the vagus nerve can cause dysphagia, dysarthria and dryness; uvula deviation (towards the contrary side of the sore); and transient parasympathetic impacts. Parallel medullary condition (back sub-par cerebellar course localized necrosis) prompts the annihilation of the glossopharyngeal and vagus nerves, the core uncertain, the single core, and the spin cerebellar parcels.

Mechanical modifications of the vagus nerve might be identified with passionate issues (discouragement and uneasiness) in patients with persistent obstructive aviation route infection and congestive cardiovascular breakdown. One of its dysfunctions could likewise be a cause of torment in a similar patient populace.

Chapter 2. Vagus Nerve Role in Intestinal Inflammation, Mood and Appetite Control

Albeit the gastrointestinal (GI) lot contains inborn neural plexuses that permit a critical level of free command over GI capacities, the focal sensory system gives outward neural data sources that balance, direct and incorporate these capacities. Specifically, the vagus nerve (VN) gives the parasympathetic innervation to the GI plot, co-ordinates the intricate cooperation among focal and fringe neural control systems. This survey will examine the physiological jobs of the afferent (tactile) and engine (efferent) vagus in guideline of hunger, mind-set and the insusceptible framework, just as the pathophysiological results of VN brokenness bringing about stoutness, disposition problems and irritation. The remedial capability of VN adjustment to lessen or turn around these pathophysiological results and reestablish autonomic homeostasis will likewise be talked about.

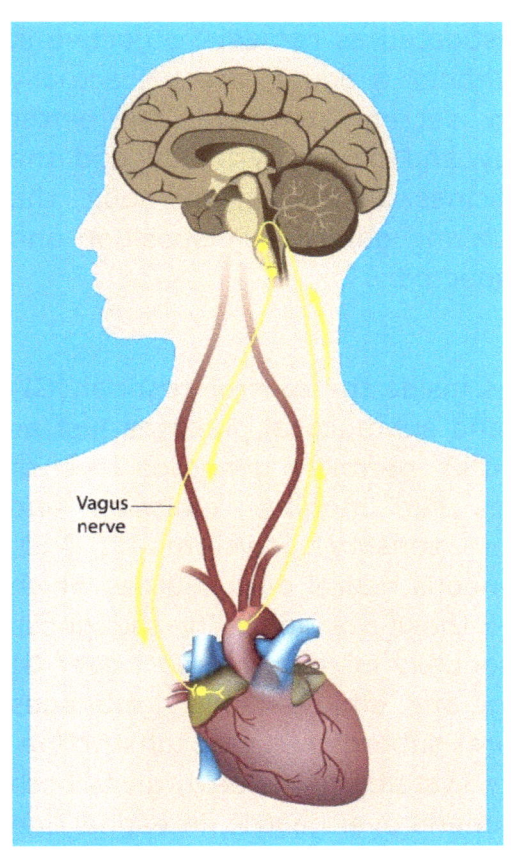

The vagus nerve (VN), the longest cranial nerve in the body, directs gut physiology, but at the same time is engaged with controlling the cardiovascular, respiratory, invulnerable and endocrine frameworks. Until now, its part in the guideline of hunger and corpulence is progressively perceived, and includes a perplexing transaction among focal and fringe systems including both afferent and efferent VN filaments. Essentially, it is progressively perceived that the VN speaks with the safe framework, for example aggravation in the outskirts is identified by vagal afferents and coordinated in the brainstem, influencing craving, mind-set and infection conduct creating, eventually, an efferent vagal sign adjusting the insusceptible reaction. The "extraordinary meandering defender" assumes a vital part in the life form homeostasis, and is at present being investigated as remedial objective in an assortment of issues. Without a doubt, the VN actually conceals numerous unseen secrets pertinent for better comprehension of physiology and pathophysiology and the improvement of better medicines. In the current audit, the current information as for craving guideline, disposition and intestinal irritation will be inspected.

2.1 Vagal Anatomy

Inherent neural organizations inside the gastrointestinal (GI) parcel, including myenteric and submucosal plexuses just as interstitial cells of Cajal (ICC's), permit a generous level of self-rule over GI capacities like motility, emission and assimilation. The focal sensory system (CNS), notwithstanding, gives extraneous neural data sources which incorporate, direct, and tweak these reactions. The thoughtful sensory system gives an essentially inhibitory impact over GI muscle and mucosal discharge and, simultaneously, manages GI blood course through neural-subordinate vasoconstriction. The parasympathetic sensory system, conversely, gives both excitatory and inhibitory command over gastric, intestinal and pancreatic capacities, reminiscent of a more unpredictable homeostatic guideline. The stomach and upper GI parcel specifically get a particularly thick parasympathetic innervation, the thickness of which diminishes as one advances distally through the digestive system.

The parasympathetic innervation to the GI parcel and pancreas are given by the VN. As a blended tangible engine nerve, the vagus contains roughly 70–80% tactile filaments, contingent upon the species4. The cell collections of these pseudo unipolar tactile neurons are situated in the matched no dose ganglia (mediocre ganglion of the VN) situated in the cross over cycle of the principal cervical vertebra, albeit some cell bodies in the throat (unrivaled) ganglion may give innervation to the GI plot. GI vagal afferents are primarily unmyelinated C-or daintily myelinated A gamma-strands and are grouped dependent on the area of their open field (mucosa, muscle or serosa-mesenteric), the locale of GI lot innervated, essential upgrade methodology (compound, osmotic, mechanical), or their reaction to extension or pressure5. Most of vagal afferents are delicate to low pressing factor expansion, albeit some vagal afferents can react to high extension pressures; while most of GI vagal afferents traffic is interceptive, accordingly almost certainly, they assume a part in nociception, or in the enthusiastic full of feeling reaction to torment.

The focal terminals of vagal afferents enter the brainstem by means of the tractus solitarius (TS), and neurotransmitter onto neurons of the core of the tractus solitarius (NTS) utilizing glutamate as their rule synapse. Some vagal afferents additionally make single reflex associations inside the dorsal engine core of the vagus (DMV), or with neurons of the space postrema (AP). Together, the NTS, DMV and AP, known as the dorsal vagal complex (DVC), work as a basic crossing point in the reconciliation of climbing interceptive signs with sliding viscera-motor signals. The whole DVC region, which lies ventral to the fourth ventricle, is profoundly vascularized with fenestrated vessels and is basically a circumventricular organ. An extra layer of sub ependymal cerebrospinal reaching neurons (CSF-cNs) are situated between the CSF and DVC neurons and may coordinate the identification of flowing signs with the tweak of autonomic, including GI, capacities.

The NTS seems coordinated in a viscerotopic way as per the district of afferent information. NTS neurons coordinate the immense volume of tangible data along with inputs got from other brainstem and higher CNS cores associated with autonomic homeostatic guideline. The coordinated reaction is then transferred to the neighboring DMV which contains the preganglionic parasympathetic engine neurons that send the yield reaction back to the viscera through the efferent VN. The NTS-DMV neural connection utilizes glutamate, GABA or catecholamine as synapses, in spite of the fact that proof from a few gatherings recommends that, under exploratory conditions, GABA is the overwhelming synapse. Vagal efferent surge to the viscera, in this way, has all the earmarks of being under a tonic inhibitory impact. Dendritic projections of NTS and DMV neurons intermix inside the different sub nuclei, notwithstanding, conceivably giving a methods by which autonomic reflexes might be incorporated across organ framework.

In contrast to the NTS, the DMV doesn't show a viscerotopic or organotopic association. All things considered, DMV neurons are coordinated in axle molded 'sections' that reach out all through the rostro-caudal degree of the core and innervate the GI lot by means of one of the five sub diaphragmatic vagal branches. In people, the DMV can be partitioned into nine unmistakable sub nuclei with six particular morphological and neurochemical neuronal aggregates. Most GI areas get innervation from more than one sub diaphragmatic vagal branch, notwithstanding; the stomach is innervated by the foremost and back gastric branches just as the hepatic branch, the duodenum is innervated by all vagal branches, and the colon is innervated by both the celiac and adornment celiac branches. In people, the vagus innervates the correct 66% of the cross over colon, with parasympathetic innervation to one side third of the cross over colon, the diving colon and rectum emerging from the pelvic nerves. Early neuronal following investigations showed vagal efferent filaments were available inside the celiac ganglion proposing a job in the balance of splenic nerves and a likely anatomical reason for the cholinergic mitigating pathway (CAIP). The utilization of the trans-synaptic, pseudo rabies infection (PRV), to plan the focal neurocircuits innervating the spleen didn't, notwithstanding, find marking in the DMV. Vagal nerve incitement obviously regulates splenic capacity, yet the anatomical and robotic premise of this activity presently can't seem to be explained. For the motivations behind this audit, the standard CNS regions and information sources engaged with the tweak of GI vagal reflexes by diet, aggravation and state of mind problems are laid out.

2.2 Effects of Diet and Obesity on Vagus Nerve Functions

The GI lot is one of a few organs that add to the fringe motioning of food admission and satiety and, progressively, vagally-intervened reflexes are perceived as being basic to the neural control of energy homeostasis especially the present moment (homeostatic), instead of longer-term (indulgent), control of hunger and food consumption, albeit plainly the two pathways are between related and subordinate.

Gastric widening enacts vagal afferent mechanoreceptors in a portion subordinate way, recommending that some mechanosensitive afferents control supper size by means of motioning of volume or burden. Conversely, chemo sensitive vagal afferents are enacted because of luminal pH, osmolality, and synthetic incitement, in spite of the fact that they can likewise be initiated by light stroking or pressure of the mucosa. Mucosal afferents are generally plentiful in the upper small digestive system, where they innervate the mucosal villae or graves. Afferent terminals are found in closeness to mucosal enteroendocrine cells and react to the middle people they discharge. More than 30 GI neurohormones have been distinguished and many assume fundamentally significant parts in assimilation, retention and satiety flagging. Most of these GI neurohormones actuate their separate receptors present on vagal afferent sensitive spots in a dominatingly paracrine way, expanding vagal afferent terminating and coming about, eventually, in a scope of instinctive impacts including gastric unwinding, diminished gastric purging, adjusted motility and pancreatic emission. Ghrelin, interestingly, is delivered from the stomach and hinders vagal afferent terminating and is, until this point, the solitary GI neurohormone that invigorates taking care of straightforwardly, as well as constricting the anorexigenic activities of CCK and leptin.

Notwithstanding being actuated basically in a roundabout way, some chemo sensitive vagal afferents can react straightforwardly to supplements; discrete subpopulations of gastric vagal afferents are initiated while hepatic vagal afferents are hindered, by raised glucose levels. Hepatic vagal afferents innervating the gateway vein are in a remarkable anatomical situation to react quickly to supplements following intestinal assimilation; their action is additionally regulated by amino acids (expanded or diminished, contingent upon the amino corrosive) proposing a nearby relationship between hepatic vagal afferent action and food ingestion.

Ensuing to their delivery, GI neurohormones enter the circulatory system from where they may likewise apply non-paracrine impacts on vagal action. In people, circling levels of without platelet 5-HT increment 3 overlap following dinner ingestion while CCK levels increment 5–8 crease. Initially thought to have a tight blood-ganglion boundary, flowing substances39 promptly access, consequently conceivably modify the movement of, vagal afferent somata straightforwardly. GI vagal afferent somata show an assortment of receptors for synapses/modulators and in essentially every occurrence concentrated to date, the activities of GI neurohormones on vagal afferent neurons impersonate those at their fringe terminals.

A few of these GI neurohormones additionally act midway to regulate the action of brainstem vagal neurons. CCK, GLP-1 and 5-HT, for instance, additionally all go about as synapses/modulators inside the brainstem to influence vagal afferent and efferent reactions either straightforwardly or by implication. We have exhibited beforehand that CCK can initiate NTS neurons even after specific careful part of vagal afferent rootlets, inferring an immediate focal activity. While the commitment of paracrine versus hormonal balance of vagal neurocircuits by GI neurohormones isn't clear, GI neurohormones seem fit for applying composed, however transiently unmistakable, activities to manage vagally subordinate capacities.

Obesity and High Fat Diet Affect Vagal Plasticity

Studies from a few research facilities have exhibited that, in the two people and creature models, the capacity of vagal afferents to react to GI neuropeptides is undermined by weight or openness to a high fat eating routine. The activities of CCK, for instance, to increment vagal afferent action is decreased in stout subjects just as people. Additionally, subpopulations of vagal afferent neurons from subjects took care of a high fat eating routine become leptin safe at the beginning of hyperphagia. It ought to likewise be noted however that, instead of the activities of leptin being weakened consistently following states of overabundance energy admission, an activity of leptin to restrain gastric pressure receptors in subject just gets evident after openness to a high fat eating routine. Such changes seem to act in show, nonetheless, to advance expanded food consumption. A few gatherings have shown that vagal neurocircuits display a critical level of pliancy and their 'reaction aggregate', is adjusted by progressing physiological, and pathophysiological, conditions. Under fasting conditions, while flowing CCK levels are low, the thickness of cannabinoid (CB1), and melanin concentrating chemical (MCH1) receptors on vagal afferent neurons is expanded; this 'orexigenic aggregate' is related with an increment in food admission. Then again, following re-taking care of, or an increment in circling CCK levels, Y2 receptor articulation increments while CB1 receptor articulation diminishes; this 'anorexigenic aggregate' is related with a decline in food consumption. In diet-incited heftiness, in any case, vagal afferent neurons seem fixed in an orexigenic aggregate, paying little heed to taking care of status, steady of an expanded 'drive' for food consumption or a diminished satiety reaction. Moreover, in diet-prompted corpulent subject, the mechanosensitivity of vagal afferents is diminished and one ongoing investigation recommended that the ghrelin's inhibitory activities on vagal afferent terminating are lost, reminiscent of an all the more wide-spread dysregulation of vagal afferents, not just a deficiency of satiety flagging. Interestingly, different investigations exhibited that, instead of losing viability, in corpulent subject ghrelin can repress the actuation of both gastric mucosal and pressure delicate vagal afferents, which would be relied upon to build its orexigenic activities.

While specialized contrasts between studies may clarify a portion of these distinctions, obviously the impacts of diet and weight on vagal afferent responsiveness is multifactorial and is probably going to be influenced by vagal afferent sort, sex, and season of day and taking care of status. When all is said in done, both vagal afferent and efferent neurons show up less edgy in diet-instigated hefty subjects; a summed up decline in neuronal volatility would bargain the capacity of vagal afferents and efferent to react to any flag, mechanical or synthetic.

An abatement in neuronal edginess is probably not going to be the sole component behind loss of vagal afferent responsiveness, in any case. Quality articulation levels of the development chemical secretagogue (ghrelin) receptor shows a diurnal beat and the mechanosensitivity of gastric vagal afferents shows a striking circadian mood, diminishing three-overlap during the dim cycle when taking care of in subject is predominant inferring that vagal afferent responsiveness to food ingestion is directed by taking care of cycles and the hour of day. This circadian reliance is lost in corpulence, in any case, working together with a misfortune in capacity of leptin to build mechanosensitivity, expanding daytime taking care of.

It still needs to be resolved whether these progressions in vagal afferent properties with heftiness are correlative or causative, notwithstanding. One late investigation proposes that, in subjects, the capacity of glucose to tweak serotonin motioning in GI vagal afferents is lost after just 3–7 days of openness to a high fat eating routine, suggesting that diminished vagal tactile flagging is influenced preceding corpulence. Indeed, even one day of openness to a high fat eating routine expands the enrollment of traditionally initiated macrophages (M1) to the no dose ganglion of subject, recommending that even momentary openness can actuate aggravation in the vagal afferent framework.

Effects of Gut Micro biota on Vagus Nerve

A critical, and developing, collection of writing upholds the activities of gastrointestinal luminal microorganisms to balance gut-cerebrum flagging through vagal afferents, the purported micro biota-gut-mind pivot (MGB hub). While gut micro biota may ordinarily be relied upon to actuate vagal afferents straightforwardly just under conditions where intestinal penetrability is undermined (for example following aggravation or stress), luminal microbes may initiate vagal afferents in a roundabout way, resulting to incitement and arrival of neuroactive middle people from enteroendocrine cells or gut related lymphoid tissue (GALT). Notwithstanding their possible part in the guideline of gut capacities including motility and emission, and enactment of invulnerable reactions, the gut micro biota have very much depicted jobs in 'higher' CNS capacities, including disposition, stress-related mental conditions and memory. Organization of Citrobacter subjectium to subject, for instance, builds uneasiness like practices in a vagally-reliant way while Bifidobacterium longum NC3001 standardized nervousness like conduct following nematode-actuated GI aggravation, again in a way including the vagus nerve. Clinical examinations have likewise proposed that ingestion of probiotics may diminish tension and melancholy. Enormous clinical preliminaries assessing the adequacy of anti-infection just as probiotic ("psychobiotic") treatments, just as inside and out sequencing of the micro biome, is needed as an issue of earnestness to additional expand on the job of the MGB pivot in a few pathophysiological states."

2.3 Modulation and Inflammation of Vagal Afferents

Vagal afferents and neurons react straightforwardly to cytokines and endotoxin, not just adding to the acceptance of fever and disorder conduct, yet additionally influencing GI capacity. Without a doubt, interleukin-1 (IL-1) receptors are communicated on vagal afferents and glomus cells adjoining the VN while intestinal irritation, set off by Campylobacter jejuni disease or intestinal control enacts NTS neurons. Aggravation, including intestinal irritation, and an expansion in coursing levels of cytokines are very much perceived sequel of stoutness. To be sure, ongoing openness to low portions of the bacterial endotoxin, lipopolysaccharide (LPS), imitates a few heftiness related results including constricted vagal afferent leptin flagging, hyperphagia, and diminished CCK-actuated satiation proposing that irritation assumes a causal part in weight improvement. Vagal afferents can react to cytokines and incendiary arbiters, yet irritation prompts neuroplasticity, including the up regulation of transient receptor potential (TRP) stations TRPV1 and TRPA175, up regulation of P2X receptors and expansion of ATP flagging, regulation of sodium particle station thickness and capacity, responsive gliosis of satellite glial cells, and expanded mechanosensitivity proposing a methods by which vagal afferent flagging and affectability might be balanced by aggravation.

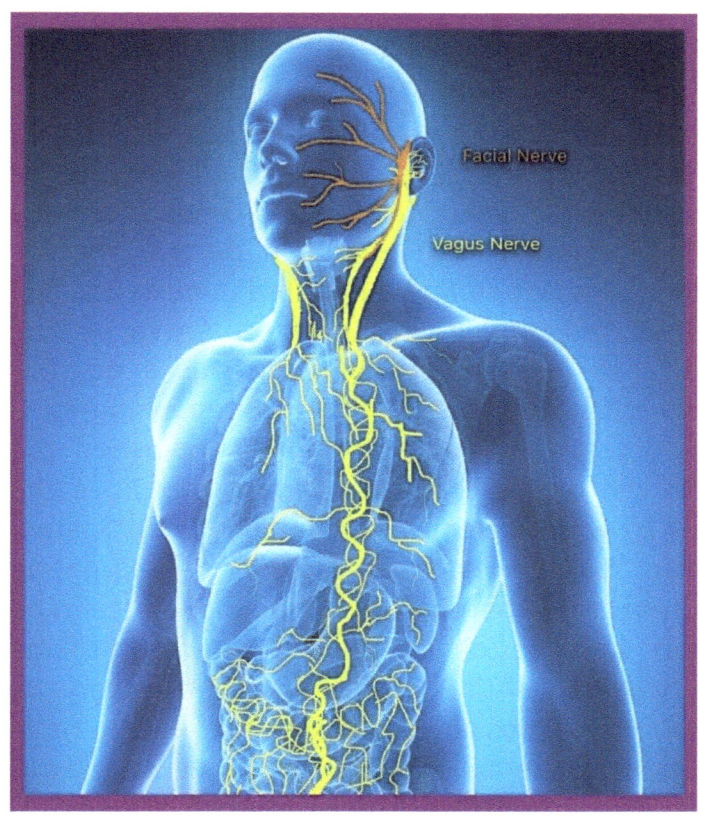

Expansions in circling levels of cytokines, including tumor putrefaction factor alpha (TNF-a) diminishes gastric motility and purging related with sickness and retching through activities at focal vagal neurocircuits. Calcium imaging examines propose that TNF potentiates vagal afferent terminal reactions, in this manner enacts NTS neurons, expands DVC microglial initiation and instigates DMV apoptosis by means of

PAR1 and PAR2 receptor actuation. Vagal motoneurons are additionally hindered by IL-1b, incompletely by means of neighborhood combination of prostaglandins, recommending that aggravation related GI problems may result, in any event partially, from dysregulation of both afferent and efferent VN. At long last, aggravation initiates DMV neurons as a feature of the "fiery reflex", which will be examined in more detail underneath.

The Inflammatory Reflex

In 2000, the idea of the cholinergic mitigating pathway (CAIP) was presented by Kevin Tracey's gathering. In a model of sepsis, VN incitement (VNS) expanded endurance by decreasing TNF creation in the liver, and particularly the spleen. This calming impact could be imitated in vitro utilizing disconnected human macrophage societies; the arrival of TNF, IL-1b, IL-6 and IL-18 because of endotoxin was altogether diminished by acetylcholine and nicotine. While looking for a pharmacological objective of VNS, Wang distinguished the alpha subtype of the nicotinic acetylcholine receptor as the principle receptor by which splenic macrophages are adjusted. In light of these discoveries, the "cholinergic mitigating pathway" was presented whereby the VN applies its calming impact by direct balance of macrophages and cytokine creation, through alpha 7nAChR, primarily in the spleen. By controlling the size of a possibly deadly fringe invulnerable reaction, this component is accepted to give an extra defensive system against the deadly impacts of cytokines. In correlation with the HPA hub or the nearby creation of calming cytokines, this cholinergic control appears to have a few properties preferring a focal part in resistant homeostasis. Thinking about the speed of neural conductance, it is fit for giving a prompt modulatory contribution to the aggravated area. In addition, as the sensory system can adjust its yield dependent on data acquired from various host locales, the modulatory impact of the CAIP isn't just quick, however coordinated as for the overall host prosperity. This thinking in the long run has prompted the presentation of the "fiery reflex".

Pathway of Cholinergic Anti-Inflammation

Albeit the calming impact of VNS is all around acknowledged and exhibited in an assortment of sickness models, the primary issue tolerating the idea as proposed at first is the missing, or exceptionally restricted, vagal innervation of the spleen. The adrenergic innervation of the spleen is more bountiful, nonetheless, emerging from pre vertebral thoughtful ganglia, especially from the celiac ganglion. Vagal efferent have been proposed to actuate these adrenergic neurons through association with alpha 7nAChR influencing cytokine creation in the spleen by means of thoughtful filaments running in the splenic nerve. These strands are to be sure in nearness to ChAT communicating splenic CD4 in addition to T cells, further described as CD high CD low memory T cells. These T cells are fairly uncommon in the spleen of guileless subject, be that as it may. By and by, VNS in bare subject (inadequate in T cells) neglects to lessen endotoxin-prompted TNF creation, while assenting move of memory T cells reestablished the mitigating capability of VNS. In view of these discoveries, the theory was advanced that adrenergic, instead of cholinergic, nerve strands enact acetylcholine delivering memory T cells, through beta-adrenoceptor actuation, accordingly hosing splenic macrophages and cytokine creation by means of collaboration with alpha 7nAChRs.

VNS of the flawless vagus nerve animates both afferent and efferent strands. Electrical incitement of afferent nerve strands initiates neurons in the NTS prompting actuation of not just the two ipsi-and contralateral efferent vagus nerves, yet in addition of an adrenergic pathway bringing about arrival of norepinephrine (NE) in the spleen and the creation of dopamine (DA) in the adrenal organ. In the spleen, NE diminishes TNF creation by splenic macrophages both straightforwardly, by means of activities on beta-2 adrenoceptor initiation, and by implication, through enactment of CHAT+ T cells delivering ACh. Enactment of presynaptic alpha 7nAChR on adrenergic nerve filaments by choline or other alpha 7nAChR agonists may build NE discharge adding to their mitigating properties. Incitement of the efferent vagus nerve hoses alpha 7nAChR in addition to inhabitant solid macrophages in the gastrointestinal lot through initiation of cholinergic enteric neurons. The invulnerable cell(s) balanced in the lamia propria, nonetheless, still should be distinguished. The degree to which efferent vagus filaments apply a calming impact in the spleen by synapsing with adrenergic postganglionic (alpha 7nAChR) neurons in the celiac ganglion involves banter since no anatomical or electrophysiological proof supporting this association is accessible. As the vagus nerve innervates the thymus, Peyers' patches and other myeloid organs, one may conjecture that cholinergic regulation of invulnerable cells (alpha 7nAChR in addition to macrophages, CHAT furthermore, T cells) happens in these organs. Under states of fundamental irritation, these cells therefore relocate, or get caught in the spleen, by means of the course.

All things considered, a few significant disparities and issues remain. To begin with, utilizing ante grade or potentially retrograde following, no synaptic association can be recognized between vagal efferent and adrenergic pre vertebral neurons innervating the spleen. Second, albeit splenic denervation and reserpine-incited exhaustion of adrenergic nerves cancel the mitigating impact of VNS, splenic nerve movement can't be identified in light of vagal efferent nerve incitement. Third, splenic nerve initiation lessens splenic cytokine creation in an alpha 7nAChR freeway. This proposes that alpha 7nAChR in addition to target cells might be situated external the spleen that move to, and are sequestered in, the spleen, particularly in states of fundamental aggravation. Taking into account the thick innervation of practically all lymphoid constructions (lymph hubs, Peyer's patches, thymus), neuromodulation may basically happen in these designs, after which resistant cells travel to the spleen. Plainly, more exploration is justified to disentangle the specific neuroanatomy of the vagal mitigating pathway to the spleen.

Another, hitherto generally disregarded, issue is the way that electrical incitement of the whole VN actuates efferent, yet additionally afferent, nerve strands prompting incitement of the contralateral vagus by means of a focal pathway. Undoubtedly, initiation of the focal finish of the cut VN apparently has similar mitigating properties as incitement of the flawless or efferent VN. Of note, actuation of the flawless (subsequently likewise afferent) VN initiates extra, unmistakable neural pathways. For instance, incitement of the unblemished, yet not efferent, VN brings out activity possibilities in the renal thoughtful nerve and enrolls an alpha 7nACh-free mitigating pathway. Besides, electrical incitement of the focal finish of the cut VN has a defensive impact in a model of renal ischemia, in any event, when the contralateral VN is obstructed recommending the enrollment of a vago-thoughtful reflex or initiation of the hypothalamic-pituitary-adrenal pivot. At long last, VNS lessens cytokine creation in sepsis by means of vagal enactment of adrenal dopamine creation. Obviously, numerous issues still need to be settled regarding the neural pathways initiated by VNS, including whether, and where precisely, the vagal sensitive spots connect with the insusceptible framework, in any event as for the spleen.

Pathway of Cholinergic Anti-Inflammatory in the Gut

As the spleen has been over and over demonstrated to be the significant wellspring of cytokine creation in states of foundational irritation (like sepsis), it is positively a basic site for neural control of removed organ aggravation. In states of more unpretentious or nearby aggravation, for example, in postoperative ileus or gentle colitis, be that as it may, the spleen isn't itself the site of the fiery affront, and other calming pathways might be included. In reality, we showed as of late that VNS forestalls irritation of the strong external evoked by intestinal control and improves postoperative ileus, an impact that is free of T cells and doesn't include the spleen. This provocative reaction was related with initiation of the NTS and DMV neurons innervating the aggravated region, viable with the presence of a designed incendiary reflex in the gut, autonomous of the spleen. This perception recommends that the CAIP may contain two degrees of actuation; the first including nearby adjustment of irritation that is free of the spleen, though vagal balance of the splenic invulnerable reaction is enrolled when the provocative cycle turns out to be more summed up.

The GI parcel gets most of the vagal efferent nerve strands and harbors the most insusceptible cells in the body. It is normal, in this manner, that the GI lot might be a significant site of vagal neuroimmune adjustment. It is impossible, nonetheless, that vagal efferent cooperate straightforwardly with resistant cells; utilizing an anterograde following procedure, we affirmed that the VN neural connections for the most part with the myenteric and sub mucosal plexuses, yet keeps in touch with the mucosal/sub mucosal or myenteric/strong organization of invulnerable cells. Talk in addition to filaments starting from enteric neurons are, in any case, present plentifully in the sub mucosa and lamina propria along the pivot of every individual villus. Prominently, varicose strands approach singular invulnerable cells intently (under 1uM) while inhabitant macrophages in the muscularis externa and the myenteric plexus are in closeness to cholinergic nerve filaments. These information show that vagal neuromodulation in the intestinal divider is circuitous, and happens through the enteric sensory system. At the level of Peyer's patches, ChAT in addition to filaments are missing from follicle and vault regions, yet are reliably present inside the inter follicular region where high-endothelial vessels and numerous lymphocytes are contained.

Prior to examining the significance of the CAIP in the GI plot, it is major to highlight that the invulnerable cell populace dwelling in the sub mucosal/mucosal compartment to a great extent contrasts from that in the muscularis externa. The last populace is less very much contemplated and comprises chiefly of occupant macrophages situated between the longitudinal and roundabout muscle layer at the level of the myenteric plexus. These occupant macrophages have a fairly tolerogenic aggregate, assume a part in diabetic-initiated gastro paresis, postoperative ileus and LPS-incited septic ileus and appear to address the guards of the enteric sensory system or the "little cerebrum of the gut". Of note, they are in close contact with cholinergic nerve strands and express alpha 7nAChRs. As with splenocytes, the alpha 7nAChR agonists' nicotine and choline hose the initiation of this macrophage populace, demonstrating that these safe cells are touchy to cholinergic balance.

The mucosal insusceptible framework is anyway more intricate, basically as the steady test by the intestinal micro biota requires an entirely adjusted balance among resilience and guard against unfamiliar antigens. One of the critical components for separation of honest and hurtful antigens is oral resistance, an instrument organized by the mucosal insusceptible framework and ward on FoxP3 in addition to administrative T cells (Tregs). We showed as of late that vagotomy decreased the capacity to foster oral resilience, a finding that was related with a decrease in Tregs in the lamina propria and mesenteric lymph hubs. Of note, vagotomized subject were more helpless to creating colitis following openness to the mucosal aggravation, dextran sulfate sodium (DSS), recommending that, notwithstanding TGF-beta, retinoic corrosive and TSLP, vagal info, or cholinergic tone, might be another major part in deciding the level of lamina propria resilience. This might be important for a few intestinal, just as extra-intestinal, safe interceded infections; diminished resilience to micro biota, for instance, is proposed as a primary pathogenic instrument in fiery entrails sickness (Crohn's illness and ulcerative colitis). Food sensitivity is another notable illustration of loss of resistance, where the invulnerable framework responds to food antigens driving conceivably to serious anaphylactic stun and even demise. In the two cases, the safe framework blows up to blameless antigens prompting extreme tissue harm, dreariness and mortality.

2.4 Preclinical Evidence of Intestinal Inflammatory Disorders

Colitis

Provocative entrails sickness (IBD) is a crippling and constant fiery GI illness. In view of clinical show, endoscopic appearance, and histology, two significant subtypes of the sickness have been distinguished, for example Crohn's illness with transmural irritation versus ulcerative colitis which includes for the most part shallow aggravation bound to the mucosa. Preclinical models give persuading proof that the cholinergic innervation of the gut significantly affects the intestinal invulnerable framework. As shown above, vagotomized creatures neglect to foster oral resilience and foster more extreme colitis with expanded degrees of NF-kB and cytokines in DSS and hapten-incited (dinitrobenzene sulfonic corrosive or DNBS) colitis. Also, subject with burdensome like conduct following ongoing reserpine treatment, which is related with decreased intestinal degrees of acetylcholine, grown more serious DSS and DNBS-initiated colitis. Of interest, treatment with the energizer desimipramine turned around these impacts in a vagus-subordinate way. Interestingly, vagotomy doesn't influence T cell move actuated colitis, demonstrating that T cells are more averse to be under direct vagal/cholinergic control. Macrophages or dendritic cells might be bound to be included; vagotomy had no impact on colitis in macrophage inadequate subject, while supportive exchange of macrophages separated from vagotomized subject or subject treated with reserpine to macrophage-insufficient M-CSF/subject created an unassuming, however huge, expansion in seriousness of colitis. These information may at any rate incompletely clarify how mental factors, for example, burdensome mind-set related with uneasiness anticipate the beginning in IBD patients. Taken together, the above would propose that the intestinal cholinergic tone, through vagal info, has a huge modulatory impact on the gut insusceptible framework, deciding the harmony among resilience and aggravation, and influencing the weakness to foster colitis.

Information on VNS in colitis models is somewhat restricted constantly to subjects, basically on the grounds that the anodes for ongoing VNS accessible should be decreased in size to be appropriate for implantation in subject. A solitary scene of VNS essentially improves oxazolone-actuated and DSS-instigated (unpublished information) colitis in subject, an impact that is autonomous of the spleen. In a subject model of TNBS colitis, constant VNS somewhat diminished sickness movement file, histological scores, MPO action, iNOS, TNF-alpha and IL-6, an impact intervened by disturbance of the NF pathway. A more articulated decrease in DSS and DNBS-instigated colitis was noted utilizing nicotine, an impact impervious to vagotomy106, and following enactment of brainstem vagal neurocircuits utilizing midway acting medications like the M1 muscarinic agonist McN-A-343, the M2 muscarinic opponent methoctramine, or the acetylcholine esterase inhibitor galantamine. The valuable impact of focal pharmacological initiation of the VN was related with diminished MHC class II articulation and decreased cytokine creation of splenic CD11c in addition to splenocytes, doubtlessly bringing about diminished preparing of CD4 in addition to CD25 T cells in the spleen. How these discoveries identify with the decrease in colonic aggravation, notwithstanding, still needs to be investigated. As splenic denervation annulled the helpful impact of focal cholinergic enactment, the creators proposed the association of a vagal-splenic nerve circuit. Of note, nonetheless, splenic denervation expanded colitis to a comparable degree as vagotomy. Given that splenic macrophages are primarily regulated by adrenergic contribution, with expanded splenic macrophage enactment and TNF-alpha creation following adrenergic denervation of the spleen, splenic denervation will without a doubt darken the gainful impact of focal VN actuation. It is inconceivable, in this manner, to take apart out the degree to which focal vagus actuation influences splenic capacity through the splenic nerve. Additionally, as called attention to before, no anatomic or electrophysiological proof is accessible to help such neurocircuitry. Direct balance of the intestinal safe framework, particularly taking into account the thick cholinergic innervation of the digestive system, might be an elective clarification for the helpful impact of focal acting mixtures, with entanglement of digestive tract or auxiliary lymphoid tissue-tweaked insusceptible cells in the spleen. Plainly, this theory, and the specific part of the spleen in colitis, require further examination. By the by, the idea of focal actuation of the vagal calming pathway is engaging and might be a promising new way to deal with treat IBD.

In models of sepsis, alpha 7nAChRs have been over and again appeared to intervene the advantageous impact of VNS. Their job in colitis, nonetheless, is fairly dubious. We showed as of late the flawless improvement of oral resistance and absence of expanded weakness for advancement of DSS-incited or T cell move colitis in alpha 7nAChR/subject, while DSS colitis was deteriorated by treatment with particular alpha 7nAChRs agonists. Then again, others detailed more serious DSS-actuated colitis and expanded IL-1b and IL-6 levels in colonic tissue of alpha 7nAChR/subject while cytokine creation of splenocytes and splenic CD11c in addition to cells disengaged from colitis subject is decreased by the alpha 7nAChR agonist GTS-21. Such contentions are not confined to preclinical models since, in IBD patients, it still needs to be resolved why nicotine and smoking is related with progress of illness action in ulcerative colitis yet has a contrary impact in Crohn's colitis. Contrasts in articulation of alpha 7nAChR, contingent upon the condition of development and the incendiary microenvironment, may part of the way clarify these apparently opposing perceptions. For instance, oxazolone-initiated colitis was related with an IL-4 intervened upregulation of alpha 7nAChR on colonic CD4 T cells which brought about a useful reaction to nicotine. Alternately, alpha 7nAChR articulation was down-managed in an IL-12 ward way in TNBS-instigated colitis and was related with a deteriorating of colitis by nicotine. How much this additionally applies to IBD patients remains anyway to be affirmed.

Ischemia

Ischemia because of serious blood misfortune, heart failure or blood vessel impediment brings about extreme cell harm and organ injury. Tissue harm, notwithstanding endotoxemia coming about because of interruption of the intestinal boundary because of ischemia, is a strong trigger for the natural invulnerable framework bringing about a foundational incendiary reaction. In reality, hemorrhagic stun increments intestinal mucosal penetrability with bacterial movement and noticeable endotoxin levels just as fundamental arrival of favorable to incendiary cytokines, for example, TNF-alpha and IL-6. Of note, high-fat enteral sustenance forestalls these changes, an impact intervened by means of cholecystokinin-incited initiation of vagal afferents setting off the CAIP. Notwithstanding its known impact on macrophages, a new report showed vagal-interceded extension of enteric neural foundational microorganisms with an increment in enteric glia and recuperation of hindrance work. In concurrence with these investigations, VNS ensured against consume instigated intestinal injury and reestablished obstruction work through enactment of enteric glia cells, autonomously from the spleen. Of note, and like colitis, organization of nicotinic agonists and focal enactment of the vagal CAIP by ghrelin and melanocortins diminishes the provocative reaction and reestablishes organ work.

Endotoxin-Induced and Postoperative ileus

Each stomach careful mediation prompts impeded motility of the whole GI parcel enduring a few days with indications like queasiness, retching, narrow mindedness to food and nonappearance of poo, alluded to as postoperative ileus (POI). Albeit some would contend that this addresses a physiological reaction to the careful affront and ought not to be viewed as a clinical issue, this iatrogenic condition is a significant wellspring of patient grimness and a huge financial weight to medical services. For over 10 years, an inconspicuous minuscule aggravation of the intestinal muscularis, set off by enactment of occupant macrophages living between the longitudinal and round muscle layer of the intestinal divider, has been distinguished as key interaction in the pathophysiology of POI and endotoxin-prompted ileus. Enactment of these phagocytes brings about cytokine and chemokine discharge, trailed by deluge of essentially leukocytes and monocytes beginning roughly 3 to 4 hours after medical procedure. As this fiery reaction significantly affects neuromuscular capacity, medicines or mediations hampering this cycle might be instrumental in diminishing POI.

A few lines of preclinical proof show that initiation of the CAIP might be an effective procedure to forestall POI. Incitement of the vagus, either electrically, by means of enteral taking care of or focal use of semapimod, all diminished the inundation of resistant cells into the muscularis, hosed cytokine creation, and improved GI travel. The impact of VNS is interceded by vagal enactment of cholinergic myenteric neurons, bringing about diminished initiation of inhabitant solid macrophages. The last express alpha 7nAChR, clarifying the absence of a helpful impact of VNS in alpha 7nAChR/subject. Of note, pharmacological incitement of these neurons with the 5-hydroxytryptamine 4 receptor agonists' mosapride or prucalopride mirrors the impact of VNS. At long last, the specific alpha 7nAChR agonist, AR-R, improved intestinal travel and diminished intestinal aggravation. Of note, and rather than the neurocircuitry proposed in sepsis models, vagal regulation of intestinal occupant macrophages is autonomous of T cells and results from an immediate contribution to the gut; specific denervation of the spleen leaves the modulatory impact of the VN immaculate, contending against the spleen as site of neuromodulation, in any event in this model of unpretentious intestinal irritation.

2.5 Evidence and Treatment in Humans

Tolerating that the VN significantly affects the insusceptible framework, one would expect expanded frequency of intestinal irritation in patients who go through vagotomy. Until now, nonetheless, strong information supporting this supposition that are not accessible. One examination reports expanded ulcer sickness, septicemia and mortality in patients that went through vagotomy following horrible injury albeit this expanded frequency of provocative interceded unfriendly results might be an outcome of an expanded requirement for gastrectomy and vagotomy in the more serious cases. One potential clarification for the absence of expanded intestinal irritation might be that cholinergic tone is reestablished by compensatory increment inside the enteric sensory system. In subject, the expanded helplessness to DSS colitis following vagotomy to be sure standardizes following half a month. How much comparative compensatory systems are initiated in different areas of the body still needs to be contemplated.

There is anyway expanding backhanded proof, in light of pulse inconstancy observing, to help an insusceptible modulatory job of the CAIP in people. In solid subjects, decreased pulse fluctuation files (low vagal tone) are freely connected with expanded serum CRP and IL-6 levels and expanded TNF and IL-6 creation in endotoxin-animated entire blood. Additionally, in insusceptible interceded infections like rheumatoid joint pain, VN action was decreased contrasted with solid controls and connected with expanded degrees of serum HMGB1, while parasympathetic tone is contrarily identified with incendiary markers (IL-6 and CRP) in patients with cardiovascular illness. At last, expanded dismalness and mortality following heart medical procedure, myocardial dead tissue, sepsis, RA, IBD, lupus erythematous and sarcoidosis has been accounted for to be related with diminished VN movement. These information propose that diminished vagal tone expands the set point of the invulnerable reaction with an inconspicuous ascent in supportive of incendiary cytokines and expanded sickness hazard.

The last proof that actuation of the vagal calming pathway is, surely, a forward leap for the clinical administration of invulnerable interceded incendiary infections will eventually need to come from clinical preliminaries assessing explicit nicotinic agonists or electrical, pharmacological or dietary enactment of the CAIP. The impact of nicotine (rectal douches or transdermal application) has been broadly assessed in patients with ulcerative colitis but with disputable outcomes. Results because of cooperation with a few nAChR subtypes and harmfulness issues in all probability forestall powerful dosing with nicotine. Enactment of the CAIP by early enteral sustenance improved clinical recuperation in patients going through major rectal medical procedure and was related with less anastomic spillage. Interestingly, in spite of should actuate the VN, gum biting neglects to improve postoperative result after colorectal medical procedure. At long last, electrical incitement of the VN, either in the neck, the stomach cavity, or the ear, might be considered as therapy for persistent provocative infections like IBD and rheumatoid joint pain (RA), or will be talked about in more detail in the accompanying passage.

VNS is right now regularly and securely utilized in patients with obstinate epilepsy, misery and headache. To this end, a looped cathode is precisely situated around the cervical VN and associated with a pacemaker. Transcutaneous auricular VNS, contrast, animates the auricular part of the VN utilizing a devoted intra-auricular cathode. At long last, the cervical VN can be animated transcutaneous by low voltage electrical signs conveyed by a handheld gadget.

VNS alludes, ordinarily, to electrical incitement of the left cervical vagus, the correct vagus being believed to be all the more firmly connected with cardiovascular capacities. While not viable intensely, long haul (9 a year) VNS has been appeared to have clinically significant results, in both unipolar and bipolar sorrow, in patients that neglect to react to different stimulant medications. The system of VNS activity to tweak temperament isn't seen completely, however since the NTS (the guideline end site of vagal afferents) ventures to different brainstem, midbrain and forebrain cores, VNS can possibly adjust a few CNS-subordinate capacities. Both creature and human investigations have recommended that VNS changes synapse levels halfway; expanded serotonin levels, expanded locus ceruleus norepinephrine flagging, adjusted NTS GABA and glutamate flagging, and improved cortical hindrance have all been proposed to be liable for the viability of VNS in treating epilepsy.

The calming impacts of VNS were assessed at first in epilepsy patients; VNS decreased IL-6 and expanded IL-10 serum levels and reduced IL-8, TNF, IL-1B and IL-6 creation by confined fringe blood mononuclear cells. As of late, a little open pilot concentrate in patients with RA gave the first proof in quite a while that VNS, in fact, can possibly improve invulnerable intervened infections. Cervical VNS improved RA infection action, decreased TNF creation and hosed cytokine creation of fringe blood. Also, 5 out of 7 patients with Crohn's sickness improved after cervical VNS and stayed abating during a half year follow-up. At long last, stomach VNS during stomach a medical procedure decreased IL-6 and IL-8 creation of LPS-animated fringe blood. Randomized and hoax controlled preliminaries are progressing in Crohn's sickness and postoperative ileus ideally further affirming the remedial capability of VNS.

The utilization of VNS in the treatment of heftiness has additionally acquired some underlying attention, regardless of proof of just a somewhat humble weight reduction; concentrates in large minipig models have shown that long haul respective VNS forestalls further weight gain and diminishes food utilization as opposed to switching stoutness fundamentally. Once more, the system liable for these impacts is muddled, despite the fact that actuation of the olfactory bulb and its projection pathways, just as initiation of the hippocampus and pallium (engaged with appointing gluttonous worth to ingestion signs) have been accounted for. More limited times of VNS have been appeared to enact the mesolimbic dopaminergic framework proposing a portion of the consequences for food admission and weight gain might be identified with actuation of focal prize pathways.

Rather than the unobtrusive impacts of VNS to decrease or converse corpulence, vagal nerve bar (vBloc), planned as an option in contrast to standard bariatric medical procedure, has demonstrated considerably more effective in initiating huge weight reduction, early and more delayed satiation and improved glycemic guideline. While this shows up at first to straightforwardly repudiate the activities of VNS to instigate weight reduction, it is maybe not that astonishing since it has been known for quite a while that truncal vagotomy improves corpulence, including exogenous (hypothalamic) heftiness in subjects and people. Vbloc utilizes a sleeve cathode that surrounds the VN and utilizes kilohertz recurrence rotating current, with zero net charge conveyance, to create an extremely confined, genuine nerve conduction (as opposed to a synapse) block, that is quickly reversible and doesn't initiate any clear nerve degeneration or harm. Biophysical demonstrating contemplates recommend that a depolarization prompted inactivation of sodium channels is liable for the nerve block in mammalian nerves albeit the commitment of afferent versus efferent VN block actually still needs to be explained.

Chapter 3. Role of Vagus Nerve as Modulator of the Brain

The vagus nerve addresses the primary segment of the parasympathetic sensory system, which directs a huge range of critical real capacities, including control of temperament, safe reaction, absorption, and pulse. It sets up one of the associations between the cerebrum and the gastrointestinal parcel and sends data about the condition of the inward organs to the mind by means of afferent strands. In this audit article, we talk about different elements of the vagus nerve which make it an alluring objective in treating mental and gastrointestinal issues. There is fundamental proof that vagus nerve incitement is a promising extra treatment for treatment-headstrong discouragement, posttraumatic stress issue, and fiery inside sickness. Medicines that focus on the vagus nerve increment the vagal tone and repress cytokine creation. Both are significant instrument of flexibility. The incitement of vagal afferent filaments in the gut impacts monoaminergic cerebrum frameworks in the mind stem that assume significant parts in major mental conditions, for example, mind-set and nervousness problems. In line, there is starter proof for gut microbes to have advantageous impact on disposition and uneasiness, part of the way by influencing the movement of the vagus nerve. Since, the vagal tone is corresponded with ability to direct pressure reactions and can be affected by breathing, its increment through contemplation and yoga probably add to flexibility and the moderation of disposition and uneasiness indications.

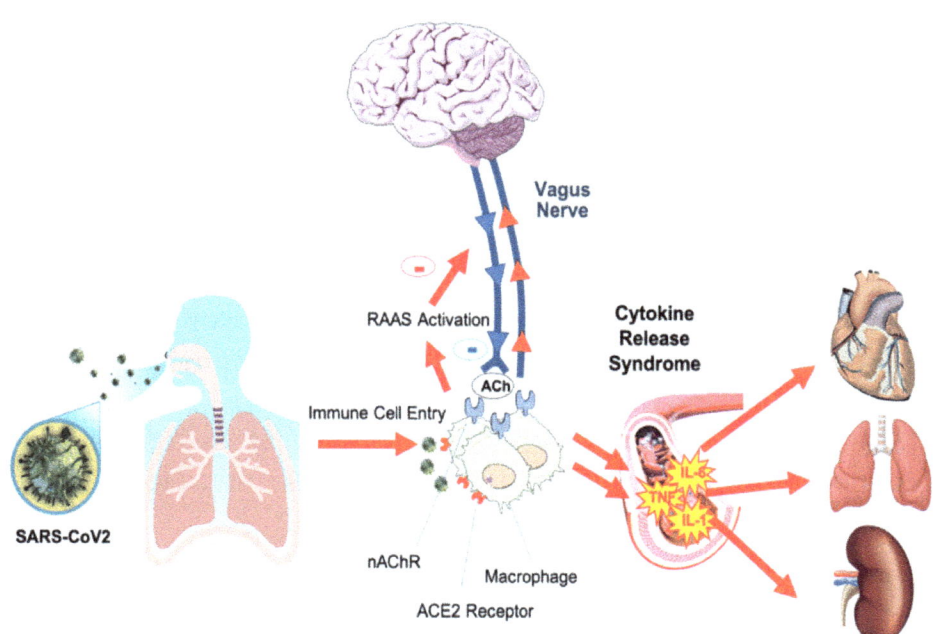

3.1 Introduction

The bidirectional correspondence between the cerebrum and the gastrointestinal parcel, the supposed "mind gut hub," depends on an intricate framework, including the vagus nerve, yet additionally thoughtful (e.g., through the pre vertebral ganglia), endocrine, safe, and humoral connections just as the impact of gut micro biota to control gastrointestinal homeostasis and to interface enthusiastic and intellectual spaces of the mind with gut capacities. The ENS delivers in excess of 30 synapses and has a bigger number of neurons than the spine. Chemicals and peptides that the ENS discharges into the blood course cross the blood–cerebrum hindrance (e.g., ghrelin) and can act synergistically with the vagus nerve, for instance to direct food admission and hunger. The cerebrum gut pivot is getting progressively significant as a helpful objective for gastrointestinal and mental issues, like provocative gut sickness (IBD), melancholy, and posttraumatic stress problem (PTSD). The gut is a significant control focal point of the invulnerable framework and the vagus nerve has immune modulatory properties. Thus, this nerve assumes significant parts in the connection between the gut, the mind, and aggravation. There are new treatment alternatives for adjusting the mind gut pivot, for instance, vagus nerve incitement (VNS) and contemplation procedures. These medicines have been demonstrated to be useful in mind-set and nervousness issues (7–9), yet in addition in different conditions related with expanded irritation. Specifically, gut-coordinated hypnotherapy was demonstrated to be compelling in both, bad tempered entrail disorder and IBD. At last, the vagus nerve likewise addresses a significant connection among sustenance and mental, neurological and provocative infections.

The vagus nerve conveys a broad scope of signs from stomach related framework and organs to the cerebrum and the other way around. It is the 10th cranial nerve, reaching out from its starting point in the brainstem through the neck and the chest down to the midsection. As a result of its long way through the human body, it has likewise been depicted as the "drifter nerve".

The vagus nerve exits from the medulla oblongata ready between the olive and the substandard cerebellar peduncle, leaving the skull through the center compartment of the jugular foramen. In the neck, the vagus nerve gives expected innervation to a large portion of the muscles of the pharynx and larynx, which are liable for gulping and vocalization. In the chest, it gives the fundamental parasympathetic stock to the heart and animates a decrease in the pulse. In the digestive organs, the vagus nerve controls the withdrawal of smooth muscles and glandular emission. Preganglionic neurons of vagal efferent strands rise up out of the dorsal engine core of the vagus nerve situated in the medulla, and innervate the solid and mucosal layers of the gut both in the lamina propria and in the muscularis externa. The celiac branch supplies the digestive system from proximal duodenum to the distal piece of the slipping colon. The stomach vagal afferents, incorporate mucosal mechanoreceptors, chemoreceptors, and strain receptors in the throat, stomach, and proximal small digestive system, and tangible endings in the liver and pancreas. The tangible afferent cell bodies are situated in no dose ganglia and send data to the core tractus solitarii (NTS). The NTS projects, the vagal tangible data to a few districts of the CNS, for example, the locus coeruleus (LC), the rostral ventrolateral medulla, the amygdala, and the thalamus.

The vagus nerve is answerable for the guideline of inside organ capacities, like absorption, pulse, and respiratory rate, just as vasomotor action, and certain reflex activities, like hacking, wheezing, gulping, and retching. Its actuation prompts the arrival of acetylcholine (ACh) at the synaptic intersection with emitting cells, inherent apprehensive strands, and smooth muscles. ACh ties to nicotinic and muscarinic receptors and animates muscle withdrawals in the parasympathetic sensory system.

Creature contemplates have exhibited a striking recovery limit of the vagus nerve. For instance, sub diaphragmatic vagotomy instigated transient withdrawal and rebuilding of focal vagal afferents just as synaptic pliancy in the NTS. Further, the recovery of vagal afferents in subjects can be reached after sub diaphragmatic vagotomy, despite the fact that the efferent re-innervation of the gastrointestinal lot isn't reestablished even after several time.

3.2 Role of Vagus Nerve in Autonomic Nervous System

Close by the thoughtful sensory system and the enteric sensory system (ENS), the parasympathetic sensory system addresses one of the three parts of the autonomic sensory system.

The meaning of the thoughtful and parasympathetic sensory systems is basically anatomical. The vagus nerve is the principle giver of the parasympathetic sensory system. Other three parasympathetic cranial nerves are the nervus oculomotorius, the nervus facialis, and the nervus glossopharyngeus.

The main capacity of the vagus nerve is afferent, bringing data of the internal organs, like gut, liver, heart, and lungs to the mind. This proposes that the internal organs are significant wellsprings of tangible data to the mind. The gut as the biggest surface toward the external world and might, consequently, be an especially significant tactile organ.

Verifiably, the vagus has been concentrated as an efferent nerve and as an opponent of the thoughtful sensory system. Most organs get parasympathetic efferent through the vagus nerve and thoughtful efferent through the splanchnic nerves. Along with the thoughtful sensory systems, the parasympathetic sensory system is liable for the guideline of vegetative capacities by acting contrary to one another. The parasympathetic innervation causes a dilatation of veins and bronchioles and an incitement of salivary organs. Unexpectedly, the thoughtful innervation prompts a tightening of veins, a dilatation of bronchioles, an increment in pulse, and a choking of intestinal and urinary sphincters. In the gastrointestinal lot, the initiation of the parasympathetic sensory system expands entrails motility and glandular emission. Rather than it, the thoughtful action prompts a decrease of intestinal movement and a decrease of blood stream to the gut, permitting a higher blood stream to the heart and the muscles, when the individual countenances existential pressure.

The ENS emerges from neural peak cells of the fundamentally vagal beginning and comprises of a nerve plexus implanted in the intestinal divider, reaching out across the entire gastrointestinal plot from the throat to the rear-end. It is assessed that the human ENS contains around 100–500 million neurons. This is the biggest collection of nerve cells in the human body. Since the ENS is like the cerebrum in regards to design, capacity, and substance coding, it has been portrayed as "the subsequent mind" or "the mind inside the gut". It comprises of two ganglionated plexuses the sub mucosal plexus, which manages gastrointestinal blood stream and controls the epithelial cell capacities and discharge and the myenteric plexus, which predominantly directs the unwinding and withdrawal of the intestinal divider. The ENS fills in as intestinal hindrance and directs the major enteric cycles, like insusceptible reaction, recognizing supplements, motility, micro vascular course, and epithelial emission of liquids, particles, and bioactive peptides. There plainly is "correspondence" between the vagal nerve and the ENS, and the principle transmitter is cholinergic enactment through nicotinic receptors. Connection of ENS and the vagal nerve as a piece of the CNS prompts a bidirectional progression of data. Then again, the ENS in the little and huge gut additionally can work very free of vagal control as it contains full reflex circuits, including tangible neurons and engine neurons. They control muscle action and motility, liquid transitions, mucosal blood stream, and furthermore mucosal obstruction work. ENS neurons are likewise in close contact to cells of the versatile and intrinsic safe framework and control their capacities and exercises. Maturing and cell misfortune in the ENS are related with protests, like obstruction, incontinence, and clearing issues. The deficiency of the ENS in the little and digestive organ might be dangerous (Hirschsprung's infection; intestinal pseudo-check), while in these regions there is less chance of vagus nerve loss.

Vagus Nerve connects the Central and ENS

The association between the CNS and the ENS, additionally alluded to as the cerebrum gut pivot empowers the bidirectional association between the mind and the gastrointestinal plot. It is answerable for observing the physiological homeostasis and associating the passionate and psychological spaces of the cerebrum with fringe intestinal capacities, like insusceptible enactment, intestinal penetrability, enteric reflex, and enteroendocrine flagging. This cerebrum gut pivot, incorporates the mind, the spinal line, the autonomic sensory system (thoughtful, parasympathetic, and ENS), and the hypothalamic–pituitary–adrenal (HPA) hub. The vagal efferent convey the messages "down" from cerebrum to gut through efferent strands, which represent 10–20% of all filaments and the vagal afferents "up" from the intestinal divider to the mind representing 80–90% of all filaments. The vagal afferent pathways are associated with the enactment/guideline of the HPA hub, which arranges the versatile reactions of the life form to stressors of any sort. Ecological pressure, just as raised fundamental pro inflammatory cytokines, initiates the HPA hub through emission of the corticotrophin-delivering factor (CRF) from the nerve center. The CRF discharge invigorates adrenocorticotropic chemical (ACTH) emission from pituitary organ. This incitement, thus, prompts cortisol discharge from the adrenal organs. Cortisol is a significant pressure chemical that influences numerous human organs, including the mind, bones, muscles, and muscle to fat ratio.

Both neural (vagus) and hormonal (HPA pivot) lines of correspondence join to permit cerebrum to impact the exercises of intestinal utilitarian effector cells, like insusceptible cells, epithelial cells, enteric neurons, smooth muscle cells, interstitial cells of Cajal, and enterochromaffin cells. These cells, then again, are affected by the gut micro biota. The gut micro biota significantly affects the mind gut pivot cooperating locally with intestinal cells and ENS, yet additionally by straightforwardly impacting neuroendocrine and metabolic frameworks. Arising information support the part of micro biota in affecting uneasiness and burdensome like practices. Studies led on sans germ creatures exhibited that micro biota impact pressure reactivity and uneasiness like conduct and control the set point for HPA movement. In this way, these creatures by and large show a diminished tension and an expanded pressure reaction with increased degrees of ACTH and cortisol.

In the event of food admission, vagal afferents innervating the gastrointestinal parcel give a quick and discrete record of absorbable food just as circling and put away fills, while vagal efferent along with the hormonal instruments codetermine the pace of supplement retention, stockpiling, and preparation. Histological and electrophysiological proof shows that instinctive afferent endings of the vagus nerve in the digestive tract express an assorted exhibit of compound and mechanosensitive receptors. These receptors are focuses of gut chemicals and administrative peptides that are delivered from enteroendocrine cells of the gastrointestinal framework because of supplements, by distension of the stomach and by neuronal signs. They impact the control of food admission and guideline of satiety, gastric exhausting and energy balance by sending signals emerging from the upper gut to the core of the lone parcel in the mind. The greater part of these chemicals, like peptide cholecystokinin (CCK), ghrelin, and leptin are touchy to the supplement content in the gut and are associated with controlling transient sensations of craving and satiety.

Cholecystokinin directs gastrointestinal capacities, including restraint of gastric purging and food consumption through initiation of CCK-1 receptors on vagal afferent filaments innervating the gut. Also, CCK is significant for discharge of pancreatic liquid and creating gastric corrosive, getting the gallbladder, diminishing gastric purging, and working with processing. Soaked fat, long-chain unsaturated fats, amino acids, and little peptides that outcome from protein assimilation animate the arrival of CCK from the small digestive system. There are different naturally dynamic types of CCK, arranged by the quantity of amino acids they contain, i.e., CCK-5, CCK-8, CCK-22, and CCK-33. In neurons, CCK-8 is consistently the prevailing structure, though the endocrine gut cells contain a combination of little and bigger CCK peptides of which CCK-33 or CCK-22 frequently prevail. In subjects, both long-and short-chain unsaturated fats from food actuate jejunal vagal afferent nerve strands, however do as such by unmistakable components. Short-chain unsaturated fats, for example, butyric corrosive directly affect vagal afferent terminals while the long-chain unsaturated fats initiate vagal afferents by means of a CCK-subordinate instrument. Exogenous organization of CCK seems to repress endogenous CCK emission. CCK is likewise present in enteric vagal afferent neurons, in cerebral cortex, in the thalamus, nerve center, basal ganglia, and dorsal hindbrain, and capacities as a synapse. It straightforwardly actuates vagal afferent terminals in the NTS by expanding calcium discharge. Further, there is proof that CCK can enact neurons in the hindbrain and intestinal myenteric plexus (a plexus which gives engine innervation to the two layers of the solid layer of the gut), in subjects and that vagotomy or capsaicin treatment brings about a weakening of CCK-instigated Fos articulation (a sort of a proto-oncogene) in the mind. There is additionally significant proof that raised degrees of CCK actuate sensations of nervousness. In this manner, CCK is utilized as a test specialist to show uneasiness problems in people and creatures.

Ghrelin is another chemical delivered into course from the stomach and assumes a vital part in invigorating food consumption by repressing vagal afferent terminating. Flowing ghrelin levels are expanded by fasting and fall after a feast. Focal or fringe organization of acylated ghrelin to subjects intensely invigorates food admission and development chemical delivery, and constant organization causes weight acquire. The activity of ghrelin's on taking care of is annulled or weakened in subjects that have gone through vagotomy or treatment with capsaicin, a particular afferent neurotoxin. In people, intravenous mixture or subcutaneous infusion increments the two sensations of craving and food consumption, since ghrelin smothers insulin discharge. In this way, it isn't astounding that discharge is upset in heftiness and insulin opposition.

Leptin receptors have likewise been distinguished in the vagus nerve. Studies in subjects unmistakably demonstrate that leptin and CCK cooperate synergistically to actuate transient restraint of food admission and long haul decrease of body weight. The epithelial cells that react to both ghrelin and leptin are situated close to the vagal mucosal endings and adjust the movement of vagal afferents, acting in show to control food admission. In the wake of fasting and diet-prompted corpulence in subject, leptin loses its potentiating impact on vagal mucosal afferents.

The gastrointestinal parcel is the vital interface among food and the human body and can detect essential preferences for similarly as the tongue, using comparable G-protein-coupled taste receptors. Distinctive taste characteristics instigate the arrival of various gastric peptides. Harsh taste receptors can be considered as likely focuses to lessen hunger by animating the arrival of CCK. Further, enactment of harsh taste receptors invigorates ghrelin emission and, hence, influences the vagus nerve.

3.3 Vagus Nerve Helps in Intestinal Immune Homeostasis

The gastrointestinal parcel is continually gone up against with food antigens, potential microorganisms, and cooperative intestinal micro biota that present a danger factor for intestinal irritation. It is exceptionally innervated by vagal filaments that associate the CNS with the intestinal safe framework, making vagus a significant segment, the neuroendocrine-resistant hub. This hub is engaged with composed neural, conduct, and endocrine reactions, significant for the main line guard against irritation. For instance, in light of microbes and other harmful improvements, tumor-corruption factor-alpha (TNF), a cytokine, is created by enacted macrophages, dendritic cells, and different cells in the mucosa. Along with prostaglandins and interferon, TNF is a significant middle person of neighborhood and foundational aggravation and builds cause the cardinal clinical indications of irritation, including heat, growing, agony, and redness. Counter-administrative instruments, for example, immunologically able cells and calming cytokines typically limit the intense fiery reaction and forestall the spread of provocative middle people into the circulation system. Further, there is a "hard-wired" association between the anxious and insusceptible framework capacities as a calming component. The dorsal vagal complex, including the tangible cores of the lone lot, the region postrema, and the dorsal engine core of the vagus, reacts to expanded flowing measures of TNF by modifying engine action in the vagus nerve.

The mitigating limits of the vagus nerve are interceded through three distinct pathways. The principal pathway is the HPA pivot, which has been portrayed previously. The subsequent pathway is the splenic thoughtful mitigating pathway, where the vagus nerve invigorates the splenic thoughtful nerve. Norepinephrine (NE) (noradrenaline) delivered at the distal finish of the splenic nerve connects to the beta 2 adrenergic receptor of splenic lymphocytes that delivery ACh. At last, ACh restrains the arrival of TNF by spleen macrophages through alpha-7-nicotinic ACh receptors. The last pathway, called the cholinergic calming pathway (CAIP), is interceded through vagal efferent filaments that neurotransmitter onto enteric neurons, which thus discharge ACh at the synaptic intersection with macrophages. ACh ties to alpha-7-nicotinic ACh receptors of those macrophages to hinder the TNF. Contrasted with the HPA pivot, the CAIP has some novel properties, like a high velocity of neural conductance, which empowers a quick modulatory contribution to the influenced area of irritation. Accordingly, the CAIP assumes a significant part in the intestinal insusceptible reaction and homeostasis, and presents an exceptionally fascinating objective for the advancement of novel medicines for incendiary illnesses identified with the gut safe framework.

The irritation detecting and aggravation stifling capacities illustrated above give the key segments of the fiery reflex. The presence of pathogenic creatures actuates natural resistant cells that delivery cytokines. These thus initiate tactile strands that climb in the vagus nerve to neural connection in the core tractus solitarius. Expanded efferent signs in the vagus nerve smother fringe cytokine discharge through macrophage nicotinic receptors and the CAIP. Hence, exploratory actuation of the CAIP by direct electrical incitement of the efferent vagus nerve represses the amalgamation of TNF in liver, spleen, and heart, and weakens serum groupings of TNF.

Vagus nerve incitement is a clinical treatment that is regularly utilized in the treatment of epilepsy and other neurological conditions. VNS contemplates are clinically, yet additionally deductively useful in regards to the job of the vagus nerve in wellbeing and sickness.

Vagus nerve incitement works by applying electrical motivations to the vagus nerve. The incitement of the vagus nerve can be acted in two unique manners: a direct intrusive incitement, which is as of now the most continuous application and a backhanded transcutaneous non-obtrusive incitement. Intrusive VNS (iVNS) requires the careful implantation of a little heartbeat generator subcutaneously in the left thoracic locale. Anodes are appended to one side cervical vagus nerve and are associated with the heartbeat generator by a lead, which is burrowed under the skin. The generator conveys irregular electrical motivations through the vagus nerve to the cerebrum. It is proposed that these electrical driving forces apply antiepileptic, stimulant, and calming impacts by adjusting the volatility of nerve cells. Rather than iVNS, transcutaneous VNS (tVNS) takes into consideration a non-intrusive incitement of the vagus nerve with no surgery. Here, the trigger is normally joined to the auricular concha by means of ear clasps and conveys electrical motivations at the subcutaneous course of the afferent auricular part of the vagus nerve. A pilot study that analyzed the use of VNS in 60 patients with treatment-safe burdensome issue showed a critical clinical improvement in 30–37% of patients and a high decency. After five years, the incitement of the vagus nerve for the treatment of stubborn wretchedness was supported by the U.S. Food and Drug Administration (FDA). From that point forward, the security and viability of VNS in sadness has been shown in various observational investigations as can be seen beneath. Conversely, there is no randomized, fake treatment control clinical preliminary that dependably shows energizer impacts of VNS.

3.4 Neural Mechanism

The system by which VNS may profit patients nonresponsive to regular antidepressants is hazy, with additional examination expected to explain this. Practical neuroimaging contemplates have affirmed that VNS adjusts the action of numerous cortical and subcortical locales. Through immediate or backhanded anatomic associations by means of the NTS, the vagus nerve has underlying associations with a few mindset controlling limbic and cortical cerebrum regions. In this way, in constant VNS for despondency, PET outputs showed a decrease in resting cerebrum action in the ventromedial prefrontal cortex (vmPFC), which activities to the amygdala and other mind areas tweaking feeling. VNS brings about substance changes in monoamine digestion in these areas perhaps bringing about stimulant activity. The connection among monoamine and stimulant activity has been appeared by different kinds of proof. All medications that expansion monoamines serotonin (5-HT), NE, or dopamine (DA) in the synaptic parted have stimulant properties. Appropriately, exhaustion of monoamines actuates burdensome side effects in people who have an expanded danger of despondency.

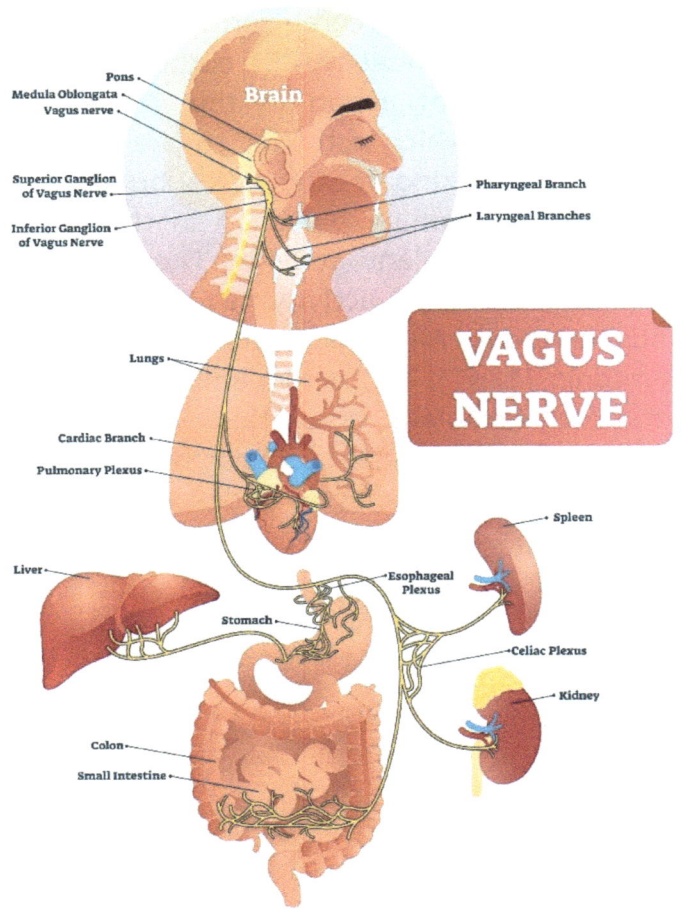

Constant VNS impacts the centralization of 5-HT, NE, and DA in the mind and in the cerebrospinal liquid. In subjects, it has been shown that VNS medicines initiate enormous time-subordinate expansions in basal neuronal terminating in the brainstem cores for serotonin in the dorsal raphe core. Consequently, persistent VNS was related with expanded extracellular degrees of serotonin in the dorsal raphe.

A few lines of proof propose that NE is a synapse vital in the pathophysiology and treatment of burdensome issues. Accordingly, exploratory exhaustion of NE in the cerebrum prompted an arrival of burdensome indications after fruitful treatment with NE upper medications. The LC contains the biggest populace of noradrenergic neurons in the cerebrum and gets projections from NTS, which, thus, gets afferent contribution from the vagus nerve. Subsequently, VNS prompts an improvement of the terminating action of NE neurons, and therefore, an expansion in the terminating movement of serotonin neurons. Subsequently, VNS was appeared to expand the NE fixation in the prefrontal cortex. The pharmacologic annihilation of noradrenergic neurons brought about the deficiency of upper VNS impacts.

If there should be an occurrence of DA, it has been shown that the transient impacts and the drawn out impacts of VNS in treatment of safe significant wretchedness may prompt brainstem dopaminergic initiation. DA is a catecholamine that generally is orchestrated in the gut and assumes a pivotal part in the award framework in the mind.

Further, helpful impacts of VNS may be applied through a monoamine-free way. In this manner, VNS medicines may bring about powerful changes of monoamine metabolites in the hippocampus and a few investigations detailed the impact of VNS on hippocampal neurogenesis. This interaction has been viewed as a key organic cycle crucial for keeping up the typical state of mind.

Serotonin is likewise a significant synapse in the gut that can animate peristalsis and prompt queasiness and regurgitating by initiating the vagus nerve. Moreover, it is fundamental for the guideline of crucial capacities, like craving and rest, and adds to sensations of prosperity. To 95%, it is created by enterochromaffin cells, a sort of neuroendocrine cell which live close by the epithelium coating the lumen of the stomach related lot. Serotonin is delivered from enterochromaffin cells because of mechanical or substance incitement of the gastrointestinal lot which prompts initiation of 5-HT3 receptors on the terminals of vagal afferents. 5-HT3 receptors are likewise present on the soma of vagal afferent neurons, including gastrointestinal vagal afferent neurons, where they can be enacted by flowing 5-HT. The focal terminals of vagal afferents additionally show 5-HT3 receptors that capacity to increment glutamatergic synaptic transmission to second request neurons of the core tractus solitarius inside the brainstem. Accordingly, associations between the vagus nerve and serotonin frameworks in the gut and in the mind seem to assume a significant part in the treatment of mental conditions.

3.5 Vagus Nerve and Treatment of Depression

Pathophysiology of Depression

Significant burdensome problem positions among the main emotional well-being reasons for the worldwide weight of infection. With a lifetime commonness of 1.0% (Czech Republic) to 16.9% (US), the expense of sadness represents a huge financial weight to our general public. The pathophysiology of sadness is unpredictable and incorporates social natural pressure factors; hereditary and organic cycles, like the overdrive of the HPA pivot, irritation, and aggravations in monoamine neurotransmission as depicted previously. For instance, an absence of the amino corrosive tryptophan, which is an antecedent to serotonin, can instigate burdensome manifestations, like discouraged temperament, misery, and sadness.

The overdrive of the HPA hub is most reliably found in subjects with more serious (i.e., melancholic or insane) gloom, when the cortisol input inhibitory instruments are hindered, adding to cytokine over discharge. It has been shown that constant openness to raised provocative cytokines can prompt sadness. This may be clarified by the way that cytokine overexpression prompts a decrease of serotonin levels. In accordance with that, treatment with mitigating specialists can possibly decrease burdensome manifestations. In line, IBD are significant danger factor for disposition and nervousness problems, and these mental conditions increment the danger of compounding of IBD.

Depression and VNS

A European multicenter study showed a beneficial outcome of VNS on burdensome indications, in patients with treatment-safe gloom. The utilization of VNS over a time brought about a reaction pace of 37% and an abatement pace of 17%. After great time of treatment, the reaction rate arrived at 53% and the reduction rate came to 33%. A Meta examination that contrasted the use of VNS with the typical treatment in discouraged patients showed a reaction pace of around half in the intense period of the illness and a drawn out reduction pace of 20% after several time of therapy. A few different investigations additionally exhibited an expanding long haul advantage of VNS in repetitive treatment-safe wretchedness. Further, a 5-year imminent observational examination which looked at the impacts of treatment as regular and VNS as adjunctive treatment with treatment as normal just in treatment-safe misery, showed a superior clinical result and a higher reduction rate in the VNS bunch. This was even the situation in patients with comorbid wretchedness and uneasiness who are incessant non-responders in preliminaries on antidepressants. Note that every one of these investigations were open-name and didn't utilize a randomized, fake treatment controlled examination plan.

Patients with gloom have raised plasma and cerebrospinal liquid convergences of pro inflammatory cytokines. The advantage of VNS in wretchedness may be because of the inhibitory activity on the creation of pro inflammatory cytokines and stamped fringe expansions in calming coursing cytokines. Further, improvement after VNS was related with changed discharge of CRH, subsequently forestalling the overdrive the HPA pivot. Adjusted CRH creation and discharge may result from a direct stimulatory impact, communicated from the vagus nerve through the NTS to the para ventricular core of the nerve center. At long last, VNS has been appeared to repress fringe blood creation of TNF which is expanded in clinical wretchedness.

Effect of Nutrition Depressive Symptoms

The gut micro biota is the potential key modulator of the invulnerable and the sensory systems. Focusing on it could prompt a more prominent improvement in the enthusiastic indications of patients experiencing gloom or uneasiness. There is developing proof that dietary parts, like probiotics, gluten, just as medications, like enemy of oxidative specialists and anti-toxins, profoundly affect vagus nerve action through the cooperation with the gut micro biota and that this impact shifts incredibly between people. For sure, creature examines have furnished proof that micro biota correspondence with the mind includes the vagus nerve and this connection can prompt intervening consequences for the cerebrum and along these lines, conduct. For instance, Lactobacillus-species have gotten gigantic consideration because of their utilization as probiotics and their wellbeing advancing properties. Bravo exhibited that constant treatment of subject with Lactobacillus rhamnosus (strain JB-1) caused a decrease in pressure incited corticosterone levels and in tension like and discouragement like conduct. It has been shown that persistent treatment with L. rhamnosus (JB-1) instigated locale subordinate changes in GABA(B1b) mRNA in the cerebrum with expansions in cortical districts (cingulate and prelimbic) and attending decreases in articulation in the hippocampus, amygdala, and LC. Moreover, L. rhamnosus (JB-1) diminished GABA mRNA articulation in the prefrontal cortex and amygdala, yet expanded GABA in the hippocampus, which neutralizes the run of the mill pathogenesis of burdensome indications: absence of prefrontal control and over activity of subcortical, anxiogenic mind districts. Critically, L. rhamnosus (JB-1) diminished pressure prompted corticosterone and tension and wretchedness related conduct. This isn't unexpected, since modifications in focal GABA receptor articulation are ensnared in the pathogenesis of tension and melancholy. The upper and anxiolytic impacts of L. rhamnosus were not seen in vagotomized subject, recognizing the vagus as a significant modulatory constitutive correspondence pathway between the microorganisms presented to the gut and the cerebrum. In accordance with that, in a model of persistent colitis related to uneasiness like conduct, the anxiolytic impact acquired with a treatment with Bifidobacterium longum, was missing in subject that were vagotomized before the acceptance of colitis.

In people, psychobiotics, a class of probiotics with mitigating impacts may be valuable to treat patients with mental problems because of their energizer and anxiolytic impacts. Contrasts in the synthesis of the gut micro biota in patients with sadness contrasted and solid people have been illustrated. Critically, the fecal examples pooled from five patients with sadness moved into without germ subject, brought about burdensome like conduct.

Effect of Relaxation Techniques on Depression

It has been shown that self-created positive feelings through cherishing graciousness contemplation lead to an increment in good feelings comparative with the benchmark group, an impact directed by pattern vagal tone. Thus, expanded positive feelings created expansions in vagal tone, which is likely intervened by expanded impression of social associations. People experiencing gloom, tension, and constant torment have profited by standard care contemplation preparing, exhibiting a wonderful improvement in side effect seriousness.

Controlled examinations have discovered yoga-based intercessions to be successful in treating discouragement going from gentle burdensome indications to significant burdensome issue (MDD). Some yoga practices can straightforwardly invigorate the vagus nerve, by expanding the vagal tone prompting an improvement of autonomic guideline, psychological capacities, and temperament and stress adapting. The proposed neurophysiological systems for the achievement of yoga-based treatments in easing burdensome manifestations recommend that yoga breathing initiates expanded vagal tone. Numerous investigations show the impacts of yogic breathing on cerebrum work and physiologic boundaries. Hence, Sudarshan Kriya Yoga (SKY), a breathing based thoughtful procedure, animates the vagus nerve and applies various autonomic impacts, remembering changes for pulse, improved comprehension, and improved entrails work. During SKY, a succession of breathing procedures of various frequencies, powers, lengths, and with end-inspiratory and end-expiratory holds makes shifted upgrades from different instinctive afferents, tactile receptors, and baroreceptors. These most likely impact assorted vagal strands, which thusly prompt physiologic changes in organs, and impact the limbic framework. A new report showed that even patients who didn't react to antidepressants showed a critical decrease of burdensome and tension indications contrasted with the benchmark group in the wake of accepting an adjunctive mediation with SKY for several time.

Iyengar yoga has been appeared to diminished burdensome side effects in subjects with despondency. Iyengar yoga is related with expanded HRV, supporting the speculation that yoga breathing and stances work to some extent by expanding parasympathetic tone.

Conclusion

While years and years prior, cutting the vagus nerve addressed a very much acknowledged treatment for peptic ulcer infection, it is presently certain that this nerve is amazingly valuable not just for the homeostasis of an assortment of organ frameworks, yet additionally for the guideline of hunger, temperament and aggravation. The remedial capability of invigorating or impeding the VN, either electrically or pharmacologically, is being investigated step by step, and the specific pathways and systems of activity are getting perceived. Non-obtrusive gadgets to animate the VN have been created, albeit the ideal incitement boundaries and the kind of nerve filaments to be invigorated still need to be resolved. Clinical investigations are progressing and will ideally before long affirm that the VN ought to be taken care of with extraordinary consideration as opposed to being cut.

The cooperation between the gut and the mind depends on a perplexing framework that incorporates neural as well as endocrine, invulnerable, and humoral connections. The vagus nerve is a fundamental piece of the mind gut hub and assumes a significant part in the tweak of aggravation, the upkeep of intestinal homeostasis, and the guideline of food admission, satiety, and energy homeostasis. A cooperation among nourishment and the vagus nerve is notable, and vagal tone can impact food admission and weight acquire.

www.ingramcontent.com/pod-product-compliance
Ingram Content Group UK Ltd.
Pitfield, Milton Keynes, MK11 3LW, UK
UKHW021446190426